# Summer Favorites

*2nd Edition*

41 Great Summer Recipes That Are Super-Fast & Ultra Easy

by Olivia Rogers

Copyright © 2017 By Olivia Rogers
All rights reserved. No part of this book may be reproduced in any form without permission in writing from the author. No part of this publication may be reproduced or transmitted in any form or by any means, mechanic, electronic, photocopying, recording, by any storage or retrieval system, or transmitted by email without the permission in writing from the author and publisher.
For information regarding permissions write to author at Olivia@TheMenuAtHome.com
Reviewers may quote brief passages in review.

Please note that credit for the images used in this book go to the respective owners. You can view this at:
TheMenuAtHome.com/image-list

Olivia Rogers
TheMenuAtHome.com

# Table of Contents

*Introduction* _____ *5*
*1. Grilled Mussels* _____ *6*
*2. Gazpacho* _____ *8*
*3. Tuna & Eggplant Salad in a Jar* _____ *10*
*4. Peanut Butter & Berry Pie* _____ *12*
*5. Plum Semifreddo* _____ *14*
*6. Cherry Bourbon Ice Cream* _____ *17*
*7. Open Faced Eggplant & Basil Sandwiches* _____ *19*
*8. Corn Zucchini Feta Salad* _____ *21*
*9. Buttery Salmon with Hazelnut Relish* _____ *23*
*10. Steak Okra Tomato Kebabs* _____ *25*
*11. Pork Chops Topped with Pickled Watermelon Salad* _ *27*
*12. Porterhouse Steak with Herbed Butter* _____ *29*
*13. Grilled Panzanella* _____ *31*
*14. Zucchini Patties* _____ *33*
*15. Chicken Salad with Crème Fraiche and Rye* _____ *35*
*16. Lobster Spaghetti* _____ *37*
*17. Melon Soup* _____ *39*
*18. Pan-Fried Shishito Peppers* _____ *41*
*19. Sweet & Savory Summer Salad* _____ *42*
*20. Summery Spinach* _____ *44*
*21. Avocado Plum Salad* _____ *46*
*22. Summer Picnic Rolls* _____ *48*
*23. Sweet Corn Soup* _____ *50*
*24. Summer Slaw* _____ *52*

| | |
|---|---|
| 25. Marinated Summer Veggies | 54 |
| 26. Pan-Fried Summer Squash | 56 |
| 27. Berry Pudding | 58 |
| 28. Corn & Cod Chowder | 60 |
| 29. Fruit Cobbler | 62 |
| 30. Summer Stir Fry | 64 |
| 31. Summery Linguine | 66 |
| 32. Summer Tarts | 68 |
| 33. Summer Garden Tortellini | 70 |
| 34. Summer Kebabs | 72 |
| 35. Squash Sloppy Joes | 74 |
| 36. Drunken Shaved Ice | 76 |
| 37. Mint Hot Fudge Sundaes | 77 |
| 38. Whiskey Wings | 79 |
| 39. Fruit Salad in Herbed Syrup | 81 |
| 40. Blueberry Banana Bread | 83 |
| 41. Frozen Peach Yogurt | 85 |
| Final Words | 87 |
| Disclaimer | 89 |

# Introduction

With summer comes a dizzyingly wide variety of fruits and vegetables. Take full advantage of the bounty with these simple, refreshing, and decidedly summery recipes.

Each recipe in this book is inspired by summer. You'll see plenty of seasonal recipes alongside some cool, refreshing recipes that will help you beat the heat.

So, get ready to take full advantage of the season this summer by working your way through each and every recipe in this book!

# 1. Grilled Mussels

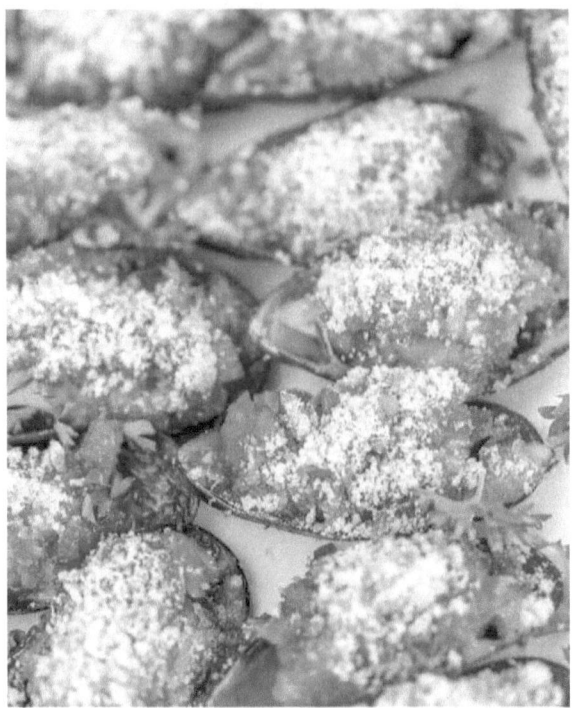

Enjoy this delicious summer dinner with a chilled glass of dry white wine.

## Ingredients

- 1 lbs. Mussels
- 1 (14.5oz.) can Diced Tomatoes
- ¼ cup White Wine
- 2 tbsps. Olive Oil
- 2 cloves Garlic (minced)
- 1 tsp Crushed Red Pepper Flakes
- 1 Bay Leaf

## Method

1. Place a large skill on the grill over medium heat. Add olive oil, pepper flakes, and garlic. Cook 1 minute, stirring constantly.

2. Add wine, tomatoes, and bay leaf. Simmer 5 minutes. Add mussels. Cover. Cook 8 minutes.

## Health Benefits of Mussels

*High in Omega 3 Fatty Acids. High in Zinc, Iron, and Folic Acid. 1 cup of mussels contains 30% of daily protein.*

# 2. Gazpacho

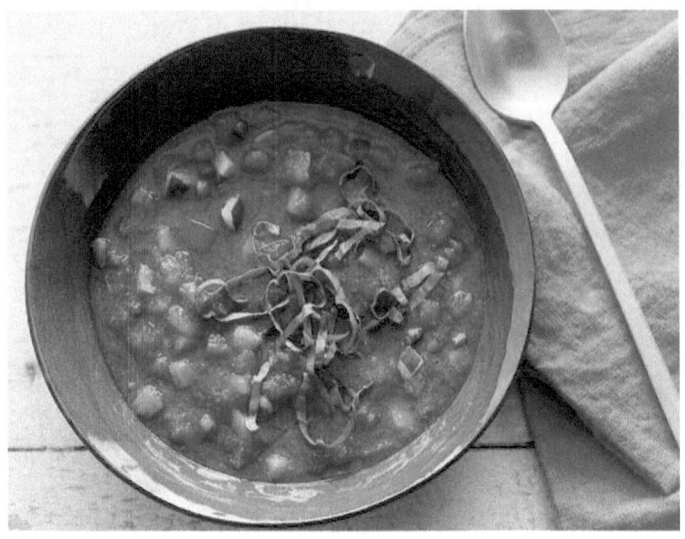

This gazpacho is the best way to cool off when you're in the mood for something more savory.

## Ingredients

- 2 ¼ lbs. Tomatoes (cut in wedges)
- 3 oz. Bell Peppers (chopped)
- 2 oz. Cucumber (chopped
- 2 Onions (cut in wedges)
- 3 cloves Garlic (halved)
- 1 ¼ oz. Country Style Bread (crust removed, torn)
- ½ cup water
- 1/3 cup Olive Oil
- 2 Tbsps. Sherry Vinegar
- 1 Tbsp. Mayonnaise
- 4 oz. Croutons

## Method

1. Fill a small pan with cold water and garlic. Bring to a boil. Once boiling, remove garlic. Transfer to a bowl of ice water. In a bowl, combine tomatoes, onions, garlic, cucumbers, bell peppers, and bread. Toss to combine.

2. Add water. Blend until smooth with a stick blender. Add mayonnaise, vinegar, and oil. Whisk until thoroughly blended. Season with salt and pepper. Chill 2 hours. Serve topped with croutons and a drizzle of oil.

## Raw Power

*This raw recipe allows you to preserve certain nutrients which are otherwise destroyed in cooking. Vitamin C is one of the most sensitive to heat so you need to eat veggies raw to make sure you get enough. B vitamins are also destroyed by heat.*

# 3. Tuna & Eggplant Salad in a Jar

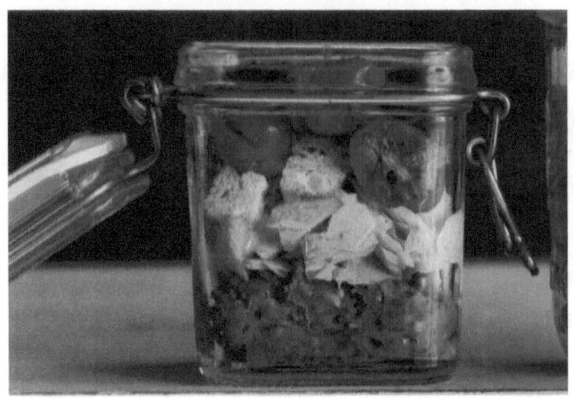

Make these hearty and delicious salads in bulk and take them with you when you go to work or out for a hike.

## Ingredients

- 2 (6oz.) cans Tuna Packed in Olive Oil
- 1 large Anchovy Fillet
- ¼ cup Mayonnaise
- 2 (13oz.) jars Grilled Eggplant
- 2 cups Breadcrumbs
- 2 cups Grape Tomatoes (halved)
- 1/3 cup Fresh Mint (chopped)
- 1/3 cup Fresh Basil (chopped)
- 2 Tbsps. Olive Oil
- 2 tsp Fresh Lemon Juice
- 2 tsp Drained Capers
- 1 tsp Garlic (chopped)
- 1 tsp Lemon Zest
- 1 tsp Red Wine Vinegar

# Method

1. In a blender, combine lemon juice, oil, mayonnaise, capers, anchovy, and ¼ cup tuna. Blend until smooth. In a food processor, pulse together garlic, eggplant, zest, parsley, and vinegar until combined.

2. In a bowl, toss together tomatoes and mint. Divide eggplant mixture into sanitized jars. Layer in remaining tuna. Add sauce from the blender. Top with tomatoes. Drizzle olive oil over the top.

# Fishy Nutrients

*Oily fish like tuna and anchovy have some of the highest amounts of Omega-3s. Omega-3 protects your brain and heart from damage caused by age, pollution, or smoke. The unsaturated fats in the fish helps your body better absorb the vitamins from the veggies in this recipe.*

# 4. Peanut Butter & Berry Pie

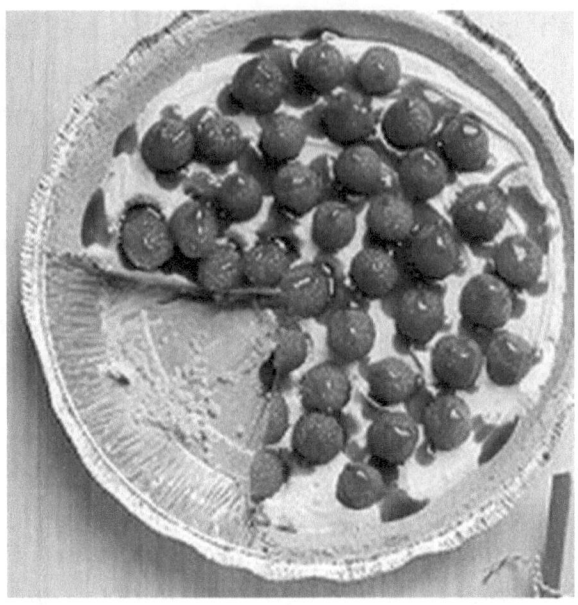

Forget PB&Js. Try this pie version of the American classic instead.

## Ingredients

- 1 Oat Pie Crust
- 4 Eggs
- 1 ¼ cup Evaporated Milk
- ½ cup Peanut Butter
- 1 cup Mini Marshmallows
- 1-pint Fresh Raspberries
- 1 tsp Vanilla Extract
- 2 Tbsps. Raspberry Jam (warmed)

## Method

1. Preheat oven to 350°F. Chill crust 15 minutes. Remove from fridge. Lightly prick the crust all over with a fork. Line with parchment paper. Fill with uncooked rice (or pie weights). Bake 30 minutes. Let cool. Remove parchment paper with rice. Increase oven temperature to 400°F. Spread jam across bottom of crust.

2. In a bowl, whisk together vanilla extract and eggs. Heat milk, peanut butter, and sugar in a pot over medium heat until steaming. Whisk constantly.

3. Whisk milk mixture into egg mixture until combined. Spoon into pie crust. Bake 15 minutes. Top with marshmallows. Bake additional 1-2 minutes. Let cool 3 hours. Top with raspberries. Serve.

## Sugar-Free Tips

*Replace marshmallows with honey-sweetened whipped cream. Find or make your own raspberry jam with natural sugar substitutes (like stevia). Make your own natural, healthier peanut butter by simply grinding peanuts in a food processor until it becomes creamy.*

# 5. Plum Semifreddo

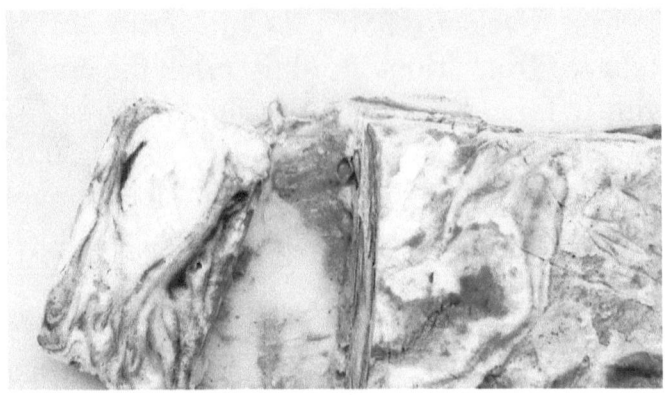

This frozen custard-like dish is a welcome sight on a hot day.

## Ingredients

- 1 ½ lbs. Red Plums (cut in chunks)
- 1 cup Chilled Heavy Cream
- 1 cup Sugar
- 3 large Egg Whites
- ½ tsp Ground Cardamom
- ½ tsp Vanilla Extract
- Olive Oil
- Salt

## Method

1. Grease a (9"x5") baking dish. Line with plastic wrap (should hang over the sides. In a pan over medium heat, mix plums, 1/3 cup sugar, cardamom, and salt. Cover. Cook 5 minutes, stirring occasionally.

Uncover. Cook an additional 6-8 minutes. Let cool 5 minutes.

2. Puree mixture in a blender until smooth. Strain through fine sieve into a bowl. Press on solids to release juice. Set aside 1 cup of puree. Let cool. In a heatproof bowl, whisk together egg whites, 2/3 cup sugar, and a dash of salt.

3. Set bowl over a saucepan filled with simmering water (without letting bowl touch water) for 4 minutes. Remove from heat. Add vanilla. Beat vigorously (or with mixer) until glossy and tripled in volume. Let cool.

4. In another bowl, whip cream into soft peaks. Mix whipped cream into egg white mixture in 1/3 cup batches. Fold in plum puree. Combine until streaks of puree appear throughout mixture (do not blend completely).

5. Pour mixture into prepared baking dish. Smooth surface. Fold plastic wrap over the top. Freeze 8 hours. Drizzle reserved cup of puree over top before serving.

## Health Benefits of Plums

*A single plum contains 113mg of potassium which you need to regulate blood pressure and decrease risk of stroke. Plums are high in fiber. Eating plums daily strengthens bones.*

# Read This FIRST - 100% FREE BONUS

**FOR A LIMITED TIME ONLY** – Get Olivia's best-selling book *"The #1 Cookbook: Over 170+ of the Most Popular Recipes Across 7 Different Cuisines!"* absolutely FREE!

Readers have absolutely loved this book because of the wide variety of recipes. It is highly recommended you check these recipes out and see what you can add to your home menu!

Once again, as a big thank-you for downloading this book, I'd like to offer it to you *100% FREE for a LIMITED TIME ONLY!*

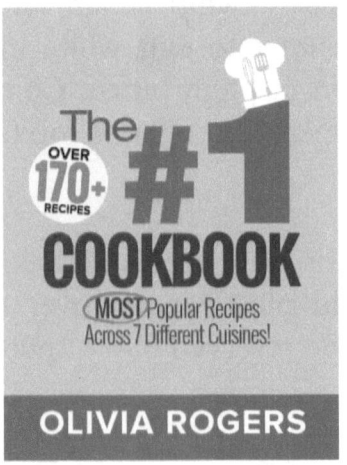

# Get your free copy at:

# TheMenuAtHome.com/Bonus

# 6. Cherry Bourbon Ice Cream

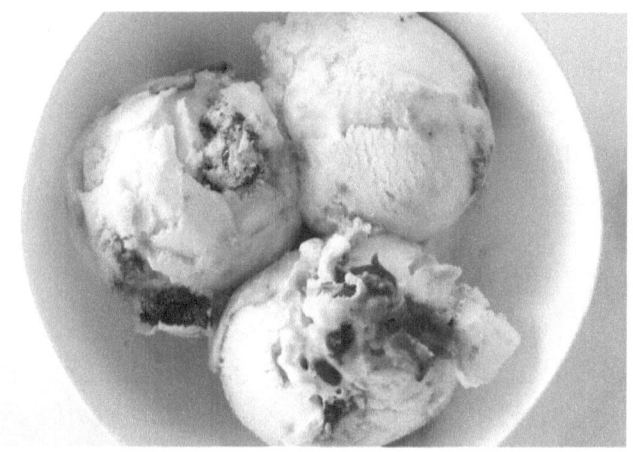

Cool down with this spiked ice cream recipe.

## Ingredients

- 1 ½ cups Dark Cherries (pitted, halved)
- 2 Tbsps. Sugar
- 1 Tbsp. Water
- 1 Tbsp. Bourbon
- 1 ½ cups Heavy Cream
- 1 cup Whole Milk
- ½ cup Sugar
- 5 Egg Yolks
- 1 tsp Vanilla Extract
- 1 pinch Salt

## Method

1. In a small pan on medium heat, combine cherries, 1 tablespoon sugar, and water. Cook 8-10 minutes,

stirring occasionally. Remove from heat. Stir in bourbon. Let cool.

2. Whisk together heavy cream, milk, egg yolks, ½ cup sugar, and pinch of salt until fluffy. Fold cherry mixture into custard. Do not over mix. Let streaks of cherry mixture remain. Chill in freezer 3 hours.

## Health Benefits of Cherries

*High in antioxidants that help prevent cancer. Helps treat pain from arthritis or gout. High in melatonin that helps you sleep better.*

# 7. Open Faced Eggplant & Basil Sandwiches

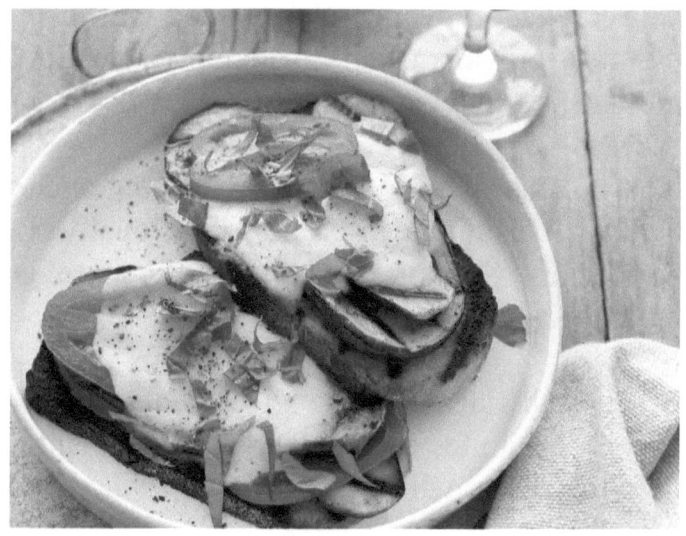

Pack these simple sandwiches for lunch or a picnic this summer.

## Ingredients

- 1 lbs. Eggplant (cubed)
- 8 slices Country Style Bread
- ½ cup Fresh Basil Leaves (torn)
- 1 oz. Parmesan (shaved)
- 1 Tbsp. Fresh Lemon Juice
- 8 Tbsps. Olive Oil
- 2cloves Garlic (sliced)
- 1 tsp Oregano (or Marjoram)
- ¼ tsp Crushed Red Pepper Flakes
- Salt & Pepper to taste

## Method

1. Heat 4 tablespoons oil in large pan on medium heat. Add oregano, pepper flakes, and garlic. Cook 2 minutes, stirring often. Add eggplant. Cook 8-10 minutes, tossing occasionally.

2. Add ½ cup water. Season with salt and pepper. Cook 10-15 minutes, tossing occasionally. Let cool 5 minutes. Stir in lemon juice. Prepare grill for medium-high heat.

3. Brush both sides of bread slices generously with oil. Grill 1-2 minutes each side. Spoon eggplant mixture onto toast. Top with parmesan and basil.

## Health Benefits of Eggplant

*Contain phytonutrients that improve circulation and strengthen the brain. High in fiber which prevents colon cancer and help manage diabetes. Contain bioflavonoids which prevent blood clots and strengthen capillaries.*

# 8. Corn Zucchini Feta Salad

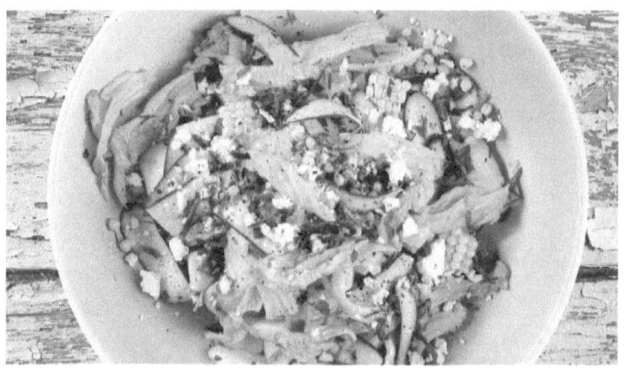

This quick salad is delicious and satisfying.

## Ingredients

- 4 ears Corn
- 4 small Zucchini (thinly sliced lengthwise)
- 8-10 Zucchini Blossoms (torn)
- ¼ cup Fresh Basil (chopped)
- ¼ cup Fresh Parsley (chopped)
- 1/3 cup Olive Oil
- ¼ cup White Wine Vinegar
- 1 cup Feta (crumbled)
- ½ tsp Crushed Red Pepper Flakes
- Salt & Pepper to Taste

## Method

1. Boil corn 3 minutes. Remove from water. Let cool on plate. Cut kernels away from cob into a large bowl.

2. Add zucchini, parsley, basil, pepper flakes, oil and vinegar. Toss to combine. Season with salt and pepper. Top with feta crumbles. Serve.

## Health Benefits of Zucchini

*High in heart-protecting potassium. When shredded, they make an extra healthy substitute for pasta noodles! High in cholesterol-fighting minerals.*

# 9. Buttery Salmon with Hazelnut Relish

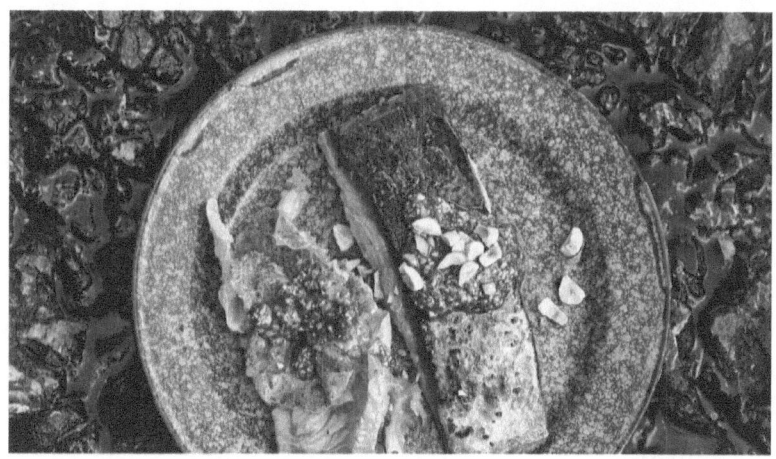

Lighten up your dinner without sacrificing flavor and satisfaction with this recipe.

## Ingredients

- 2 small heads Lettuce
- 1 cup Fresh Cilantro
- ½ cup Fresh Parsley
- 4 (6oz.) Salmon Fillets (with skin)
- ½ cup Blanched Hazelnuts
- ½ cup Olive Oil
- 2 Tbsps. Butter
- 1 Tbsp. Olive Oil
- 1 Tbsp. Capers
- 1 clove Garlic (chopped)
- 1 tsp Lemon Zest
- Salt to taste

## Method

1. Preheat oven to 400°F. Arrange hazelnuts on rimmed baking sheet. Bake 6-8 minutes, tossing occasionally. Let cool. In a processor, pulse together parsley, cilantro, garlic, lemon zest, capers, and ¼ cup hazelnuts.

2. Gradually add olive oil while still pulsing. Season with salt. Transfer to bowl. Add remaining hazelnuts to processor. Chop coarsely. Heat oil in a large (ovenproof) pan on medium-high heat. Lightly salt salmon. Cook skin side down 4 minutes.

3. Add butter to pan. Cook 1-minute, basting salmon constantly. Transfer pan to oven. Roast 3 minutes, basting once. Serve salmon skin side up. Top with lettuce, cilantro mixture and chopped hazelnuts.

## Health Benefits of Hazelnuts

*High in muscle-building magnesium. 1 cup of hazelnuts contains more than 80% of your daily Vitamin E (which maintains your skin's youthful glow). High in energizing and rejuvenating B vitamins.*

# 10. Steak Okra Tomato Kebabs

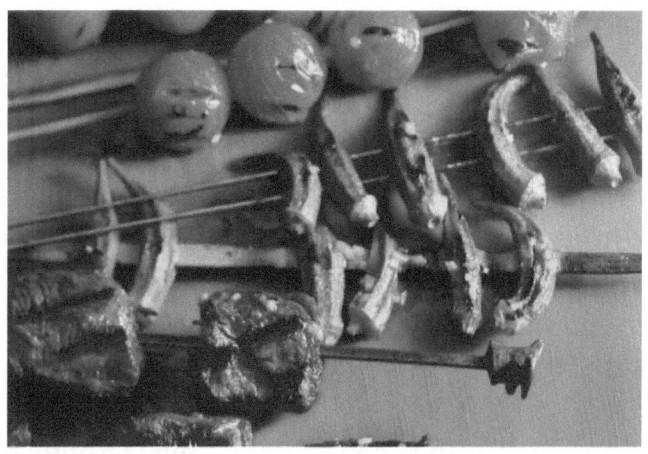

These quick kebabs are perfect for spontaneous backyard parties.

## Ingredients

- ¾ lbs. Okra
- 1 lbs. Small Tomatoes
- 2 lbs. Boneless Chuck Blade Steak (trimmed, cubed)
- ½ cup Olive Oil
- 3 Tbsps. Shallot (chopped)
- 3 Tbsps. Red Wine Vinegar
- 2 tsp Dijon Mustard
- ½ tsp Sugar
- 16 metal skewers

## Method

1. In a bowl, blend mustard, vinegar, shallots, sugar, salt and pepper. Slowly drizzle in oil, whisking

constantly. Rub steak with ½ teaspoon salt. Place in Ziploc bag with 6 tablespoons oil-vinegar mixture. Toss to coat. Marinate 2 hours. Chill remaining oil-vinegar mixture. Prepare grill for medium-high heat.

2. In a bowl, toss okra and tomatoes with 3 tablespoons oil and ¼ teaspoon salt. Place all the tomatoes onto skewers (lining up full skewers with just tomatoes). Pierce a skewer through each end of 1 okra. Add the remaining okra pierces onto the pair of skewers. Set aside.

3. Chop steak into pieces. Places pieces onto skewers. Grill steak skewers 5 minutes, turning once. Transfer to platter. Drizzle with some oil-vinegar mixture. Grill okra and tomato skewers 8 minutes. Transfer to steak platter. Serve with remaining oil-vinegar mixture.

## Health Benefits of Okra

*Helps stabilize blood sugar. May help prevent asthma attacks. Reduces acne outbreaks.*

# 11. Pork Chops Topped with Pickled Watermelon Salad

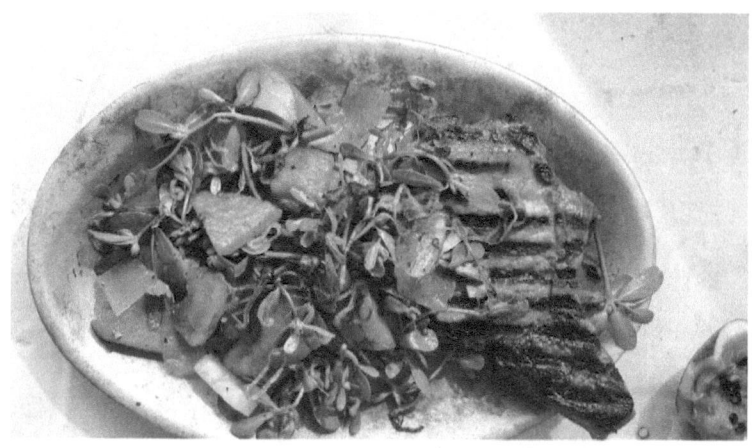

Pickled watermelon salad puts a unique twist on this pork chop dinner.

## Ingredients

- 4 Bone-In Pork Chops
- 2 Shallots (sliced into rings)
- ¼ cup Low Sodium Soy Sauce
- 2 Tbsps. Fish Sauce
- 2 Tbsps. Sugar
- 1 tsp Sriracha Sauce
- ½ cup Pickled Watermelon Rind (sliced)
- ½ lbs. Watermelon Flesh (seeded, cubed)
- 4 cups Arugula
- 4 Shallots (sliced)
- 6 Tbsps. Olive Oil
- 1 Tbsp. Rice Vinegar
- 1 tsp Low Sodium Soy Sauce

- ¼ tsp Sugar
- Salt & Pepper to taste

## Method

1. In a baking dish, blend together fish sauce, soy sauce, Sriracha, sugar, and shallots. Add pork chops. Turn to coat. Cover. Chill 1 hour, turning occasionally. Heat 4 tablespoons oil in a small pan on medium heat. Add shallots (from pork marinade) to pan. Cook 4 minutes. Drain on paper towels.

2. In a bowl, whisk together remaining oil with soy sauce, vinegar, and sugar. Season with salt and pepper. Add watermelon and pickled watermelon rind. Toss to coat. Prepare grill for medium-high heat. Remove pork chops from marinade. Grill 3 minutes per side. Top with fried shallots. Serve with watermelon salad.

## Health Benefits of Watermelon Rinds

*Contains immune system-boosting citrulline. Eaten before a workout, can help prevent muscle fatigue and improve endurance. May help with erectile dysfunction.*

# 12. Porterhouse Steak with Herbed Butter

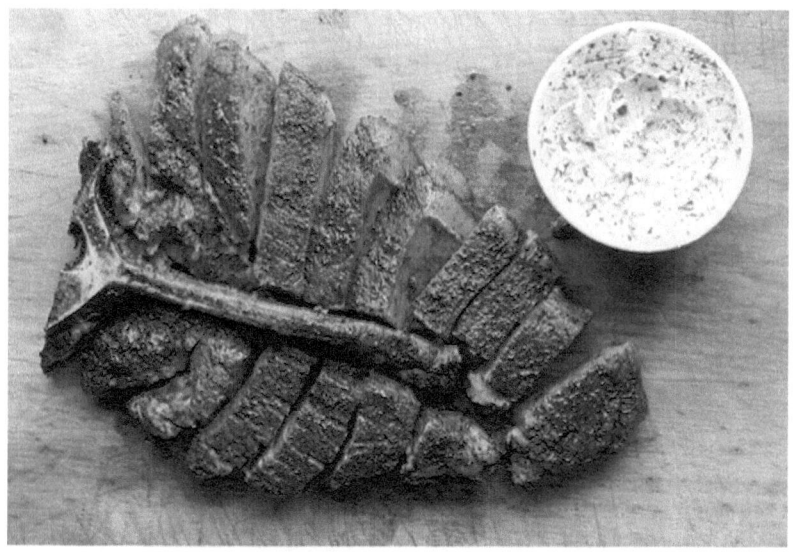

This simple dish embraces the natural flavors of each ingredient.

## Ingredients

- 2 Porterhouse Steaks
- 2 Tbsps. Olive Oil
- 2 Tbsps. Butter
- ¼ cup Mixed Fresh Herbs (your preference)
- ½ cup Butter
- Salt & Pepper to taste

## Method

1. Let steak sit out at room temperature 30 minutes. In a bowl, stir together butter and herbs with wooden spoon. Season with salt and pepper. Cover with

plastic wrap. Chill at least 1 hour. Preheat oven to 350°F. Pat steaks dry. Season with salt and pepper.

2. Heat 1 tablespoon oil in pan on medium-heat. When oil smokes, add steak. Cook 3 minutes per side. Melt 1 tablespoon butter in pan. Spoon over steak. Remove from pan. Set aside. Repeat for second steak.

3. Place steaks on rimmed baking sheet with a wire rack. Bake until meat thermometer reads 120°-125°F. Transfer to wooden board. Let rest 10 minutes. Serve with herbed butter.

## Health Benefits of Fresh Herbs

*Fresh rosemary improves concentration and memory. Fresh parsley helps prevent breast cancer. Fresh mint relives symptoms of irritable bowel syndrome.*

# 13. Grilled Panzanella

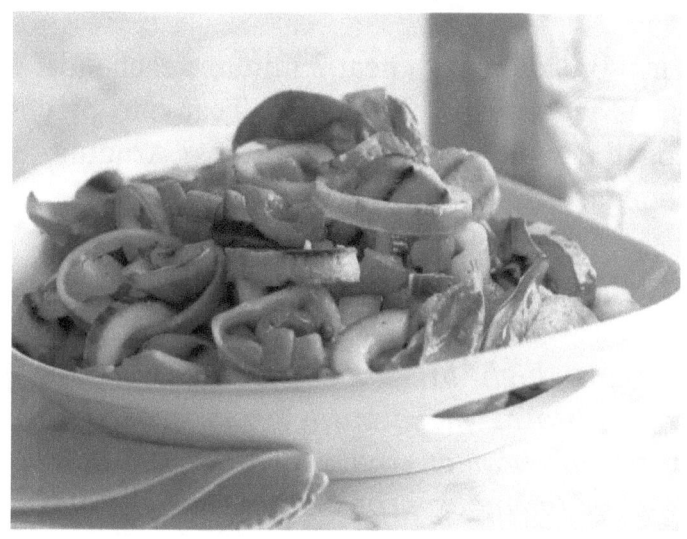

This hearty grilled salad can hold its own at any barbecue.

## Ingredients

- 1 lbs. Cherry Tomatoes (grilled)
- 1 bunch Scallions
- 1 clove Garlic (halved)
- 2 cups Arugula
- 2 Tbsps. Olive Oil
- 2 Tbsps. Red Wine Vinegar
- Salt & Pepper to taste
- 4 thick slices Country Style Bread (crust removed)

## Method

1. In a bowl, toss together scallions, oil, salt and pepper. Grill on high heat 4 minutes, turning

occasionally. Let cool. Chop. Brush both sides of each bread slice generously with oil.

2. Grill bread on high heat 2 minutes each side. Rub all sides vigorously with garlic. Tear into pieces. Toss together with tomatoes, scallions, Arugula, oil, and vinegar.

## Health Benefits of Tomatoes

*Tomatoes are high in cancer-fighting lycopene (which your body absorbs more easily from cooked tomatoes). Lycopene helps protect your skin from sun damage. The vitamin A in tomatoes protects your eyes from macular degeneration.*

# 14. Zucchini Patties

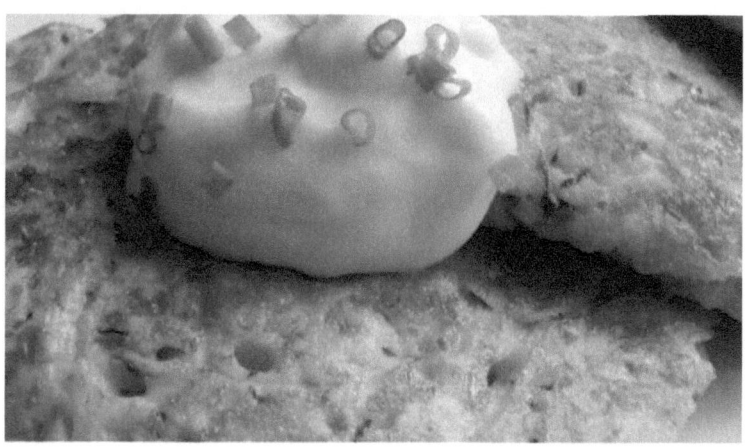

These patties are the best way to sneak a serving of veggies onto your dinner plate.

## Ingredients

- 4 medium Zucchini (grated)
- 1 Onion (grated)
- 1 leek (chopped)
- 2 large Eggs (beaten)
- 1/3 cup Breadcrumbs
- 1 ½ cups Vegetable Oil
- 1 Tbsp. Thyme
- Salt & Pepper to taste
- Roasted Red Pepper Labneh

## Method

1. In a bowl, combine zucchini, onion, and 3 teaspoons salt. Toss to coat. Let sit 10 minutes. Place zucchini

mixture in a paper towel and squeeze to wring out juice. Transfer to a new bowl. Add leek, breadcrumbs, egg, and thyme. Season with pepper.

2. Heat oil in a deep pan on medium heat. Drop spoonsful of zucchini mix into hot oil. Gently flatten with spoon. Cook 3 minutes per side. Drain on paper towels. Serve with labneh.

## More Health Benefits of Zucchini

*High fiber content helps control appetite and improve digestion. The fiber also helps sweep toxins out of your body. B vitamins, zinc, and magnesium help your body break down blood sugars.*

# 15. Chicken Salad with Crème Fraiche and Rye

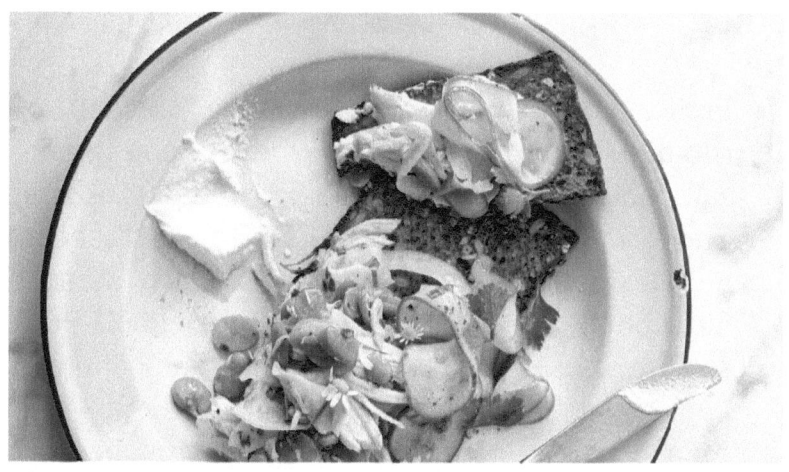

This chicken salad is beautifully accented with crème fraiche and summery flavors.

## Ingredients

- 12-14 oz. Bone-In Chicken Breast
- 4 Tbsps. Olive Oil
- ¾ cup Fava Beans (fresh)
- ½ bulb Fennel (sliced)
- 1 Scallion (sliced)
- ½ cup Crème Fraiche
- ½ Cucumber (thinly sliced lengthwise)
- ¼ cup Fresh Parsley
- 1 Tbsp. Sherry Vinegar
- 2 Tbsps. Fresh Tarragon (chopped)
- ½ tsp Lemon Zest
- 2 tsp Fresh Lemon Juice

- 8 slices Rye Bread
- Salt & Pepper to taste

## Method

1. Preheat oven to 425°F. Arrange chicken on a rimmed baking sheet. Rub with 1 tablespoon oil, salt, and pepper. Roast 25-30 minutes. Let cool. Shred into bite-sized chunks. Boil fava beans 4 minutes. Drain. Transfer to bowl of ice water. In a large bowl, toss together fava beans, fennel, chicken, scallions, tarragon, oil, vinegar, salt and pepper.

2. In a separate bowl, whisk crème fraiche to soft peaks (fluffy). Sprinkle in salt. In a third bowl, toss together cucumber, parsley, lemon zest, and lemon juice. Season with salt and pepper. Divide chicken salad and cucumber mixture into bowls. Add a dollop of crème fraiche. Serve with bread.

## Health Benefits of Fava Beans

*High in bone-strengthening phosphorous. High in heart-protecting magnesium and potassium. High in immune-boosting folate.*

# 16. Lobster Spaghetti

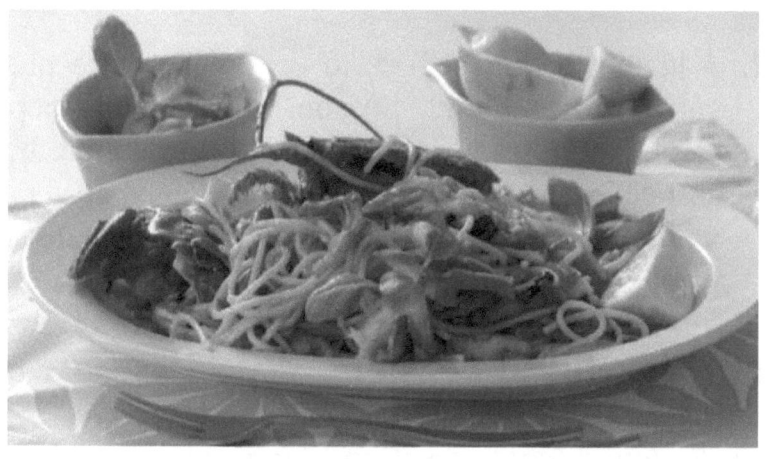

Upgrade your spaghetti dinner with lobster.

## Ingredients

- 12 oz. Spaghetti
- 1 lbs. Lobster Meat (cooked)
- 1 lbs. Cherry Tomatoes (halved)
- 1 Shallot (chopped)
- 2 Tbsps. Olive Oil
- 2 Tbsps. Butter
- 1 tsp Lemon Zest
- 1 tsp. Crushed Red Pepper Flakes
- Salt & Pepper to taste

## Method

1. Cook spaghetti until al dente. Drain. Reserve 1 cup liquid. Heat oil and butter in a large pan on medium-high heat. Add shallot and pepper flakes. Cook 2

minutes, stirring often. Add tomatoes. Cook 5-8 minutes, stirring often.

2. Add lobster meat. Toss to coat. Add pasta plus ½ cup reserved liquid. Season with salt and pepper. Cook 2 minutes, tossing constantly. Add more liquid as needed to thicken sauce and evenly coat pasta. Divide onto plates. Garnish with lemon zest and wedges.

## Health Benefits of Lobster

*Naturally low in cholesterol and high in protein. High in thyroid-boosting selenium which helps control weight. Helps lower blood pressure.*

# 17. Melon Soup

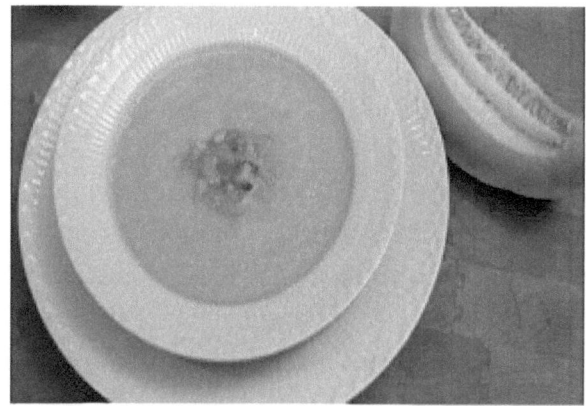

Melons turn this soup into a refreshing and smooth meal.

## Ingredients

- 4 oz. Silken Tofu
- ¼ cup White Soy Sauce
- 6 lbs. Melons (very ripe)
- ¼ cup Almond Oil
- ¼ cup Toasted Almonds
- 1 Onion (sliced)
- 10 Tbsps. Butter
- Sherry Vinegar
- Fresh Herb Blend (your preference)
- Salt to taste

## Method

1. Press tofu through a fine sieve into a bowl. Stir in soy sauce. Cover and chill. Scoop out 18 melon balls into a bowl. Season with salt and vinegar. Toss

gently. Let stand 30 minutes. Drain. Transfer to a new bowl. Set aside. Cut rind from remaining melon. Chop flesh into 2" cubes.

2. Melt 6 tablespoons butter in a large pot on medium-low heat. Add onion. Cook 10 minutes, stirring often. Cut out a piece of parchment paper large enough to cover the opening of the pot. Add melon cubes to pot along with remaining butter. Cover with parchment paper. Simmer 15 minutes, stirring occasionally. Remove from heat. Let cool 5 minutes.

3. Puree soup into blender until smooth. Cover and chill 4 hours. Ladle soup into chilled bowls. Dollop tofu mixture on top. Garnish with toasted almonds, fresh herbs, and melon balls. Drizzle with almond oil.

## Health Benefits of Melons

*High in Vitamin A which is good for skin, hair, teeth, nails and eyes. Helps improve metabolism. Acts as a natural anti-inflammatory.*

# 18. Pan-Fried Shishito Peppers

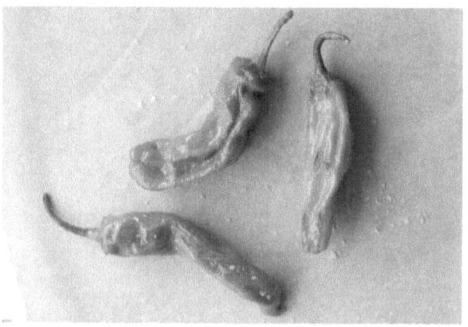

This elegantly simple side dish will pair perfectly with steak, pork, poultry, or fish.

## Ingredients

- Shishito Peppers
- Olive Oil
- Fresh Lemon Juice
- Salt

## Method

1. Heat oil in a large pan on medium heat. Add peppers. Cook 10-15 minutes, tossing frequently. Remove from heat. Sprinkle in salt. Drizzle in lemon. Toss to coat.

## Health Benefits of Shishito Peppers

*High in cancer-fighting antioxidants. Boost immune system function. Act as natural anti-inflammatory.*

# 19. Sweet & Savory Summer Salad

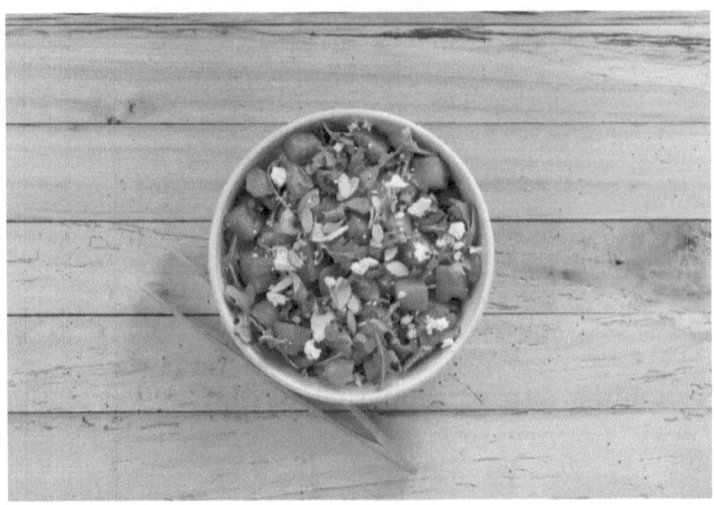

This salad combines the perfect balance of hearty protein and fruity notes.

## Ingredients

- 10 large Eggs
- 1/3 cup Flour
- 1 cup Lemon Vinaigrette
- 1-quart Vegetable Oil
- ¾ cup Raw Shelled Pistachios
- 8 small Apricots (pitted, diced)
- 1 ¼ cup Mixed Fresh Herbs (your preference)
- 4 cups Arugula
- 2/3 cup Blanched Whole Almonds (ground)
- 2/3 cup Parmesan (grated)
- 1 cup Breadcrumbs
- Salt & Pepper to taste

# Method

1. Prepare a large bowl with ice water. Set aside. Bring water to a boil. Add 8 eggs. Reduce heat. Simmer 6 minutes. Transfer eggs to ice water. Let stand 5 minutes. Peel. Set aside. In a bowl, whisk together flour, salt, and pepper. In another bowl, beat together 2 eggs with 2 tablespoons water.

2. In a third bowl, blend breadcrumbs, ground almonds, parmesan, salt and pepper. Roll boiled eggs in flour mixture one at a time. Dip into breadcrumb mixture and then egg mixture. Repeat step. Place coated eggs on baking sheet and chill in fridge 30 minutes.

3. In a large bowl, toss together ½ cup pistachios, ½ cup apricots, herbs, and arugula. Heat 3" oil in a large pan on high heat. Carefully fry eggs 1-2 minutes per side. Drain on paper towels. Drizzle vinaigrette over salad. Toss to coat. Divide salad into 8 bowls. Garnish with remaining pistachios and apricots and 1 egg (sliced).

# Health Benefits of Arugula

*High in brain-boosting folate. High in fiber which controls appetite, improves digestion, and detoxes the body. High in bone-strengthening Vitamin K.*

## 20. Summery Spinach

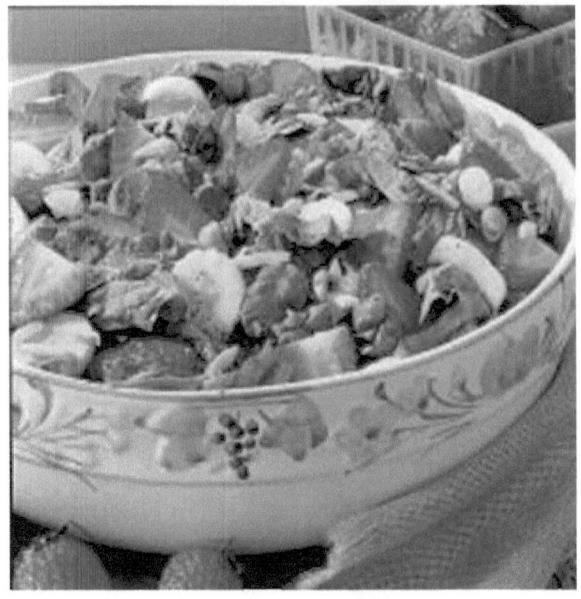

Spinach is the star of this simple side dish.

## Ingredients

- 4 large bunches Fresh Spinach
- 2 cloves Garlic (halved)
- Olive Oil
- ½ Lemon
- Salt to taste

## Method

1. Heat oil in a large pot over medium-high heat. Add garlic. Stir 1 minute. Remove garlic. Add spinach. Salt to taste.

2. Cut leaves with scissors as they wilt. Once wilted, arrange spinach on a platter. Drizzle lemon juice over.

## Health Benefits of Spinach

*Cooking spinach removes the oxalic acid which prevents your body from absorbing the high calcium and iron contents found in the leaves. A diet with lots of spinach helps relieve itchy or dry skin. Spinach helps treat constipation and prevent ulcers.*

# 21. Avocado Plum Salad

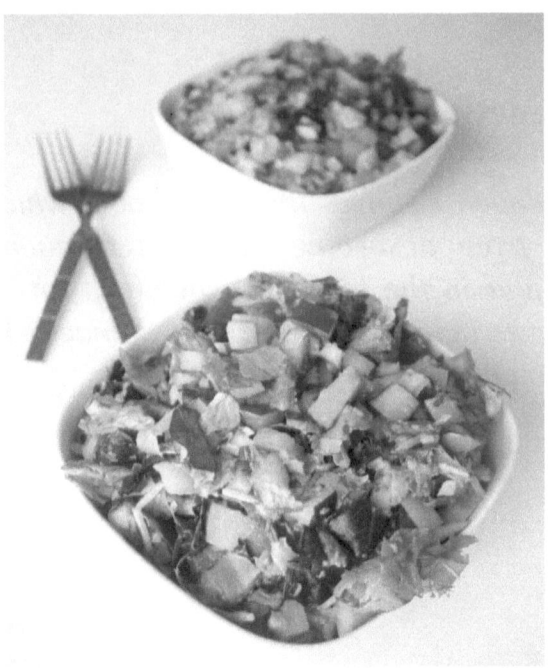

Avocado and plum bring the best of both worlds into this salad.

## Ingredients

- 2 Ripe Hass Avocados (pitted, peeled, chopped)
- 5 Ripe Black Plums (pitted, chopped)
- 1 cup Fresh Cilantro (chopped)
- 1 Lemon
- 1 Red Chili Pepper (dried, chopped)
- 1 clove Garlic (minced)
- ½ cup Olive Oil
- Salt to taste

## Method

1. In a bowl, carefully combine plum and avocado. Do not mix too much (or avocado will get mushy). Squeeze lemon juice over and sprinkle with salt.

2. Smash garlic together with salt to form a paste. Add chili pepper. Continue to crush. Add cilantro. Continue crushing. Whisk in olive oil. Drizzle dressing over the plum and avocado.

## Health Benefits of Avocados

*High in unsaturated fats that help control appetite, hydrate skin, and absorb nutrients. Avocados contain more potassium than bananas. Help lower cholesterol.*

## 22. Summer Picnic Rolls

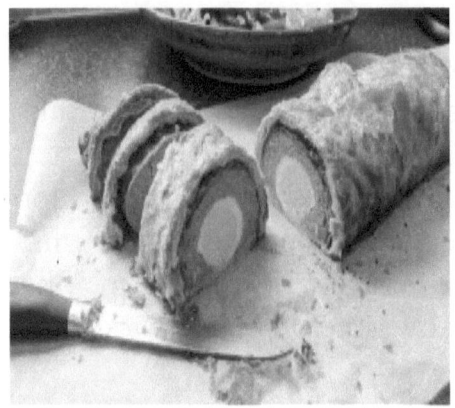

These simple little treats are the perfect dish to pack for a picnic.

## Ingredients

- 1 oz. Cellophane Noodles
- 1 lbs. Ground Turkey Breast (extra lean)
- 2 large Egg Whites (beaten)
- 1 cup Scallions (chopped)
- ½ cup Shiitake Mushrooms (chopped)
- 1 cup Canned Mung Bean Sprouts (drained)
- 9 (8") sheets Rice Paper
- ½ Red Bell Pepper (thinly sliced)
- ½ Green Bell Pepper (thinly sliced)
- 2 tsp Olive Oil
- 1 tsp Sugar
- 1 tsp Fish Sauce
- 1 tsp Oyster Sauce
- ¼ tsp Pepper

## Method

1. Boil noodles for 3 minutes. Drain. Set aside. In a bowl, mix together turkey, fish sauce, egg whites, oyster sauce, mushrooms, scallions, sugar, and pepper. Heat oil in a large pan on medium-high heat. Cook turkey mixture 7 minutes, stir to crumble. Remove from heat.

2. Push turkey to one side. Add pepper to other side. Soak rice paper in a bowl of warm water 10-15 seconds for each piece. Lay flat. Evenly distribute all ingredients onto each paper. Fold bottom edge up. Fold in the sides. Roll up toward the top edge.

## Health Benefits of Mung Bean Sprouts

*High in fiber. High in vitamin C. High in vitamin K.*

# 23. Sweet Corn Soup

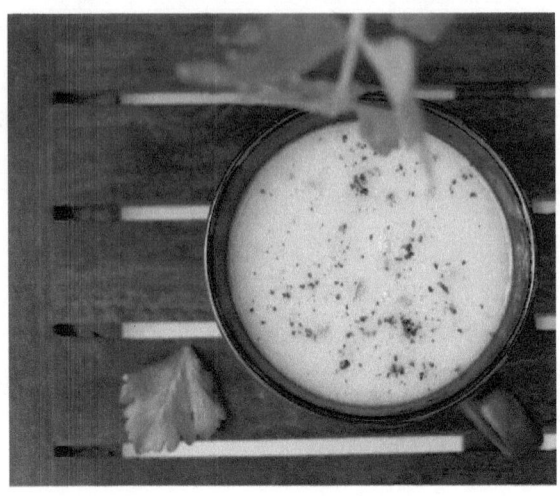

This sweet corn soup can stand alone or be paired with fresh fish tacos.

## Ingredients

- 2 quarts Vegetable Stock
- 6 ears Sweet Corn
- 2 large Onions (diced)
- 4 large stalks Celery (sliced)
- 1 ½ lbs. Potatoes (diced)
- 1 ½ cups Whole Milk
- ½ cup Fresh Parsley (chopped)
- 3 Tbsps. Olive Oil
- 1 tsp Cayenne Pepper
- 1 tsp Ground Coriander
- ½ tsp Paprika
- Salt & Pepper to taste

## Method

1. In a large pot, bring stock to a boil. Reduce heat. Let simmer. Place the corn cobs in the pot. Simmer 20 minutes. Heat oil in a large pan over medium heat. Add onions. Cook 3 minutes. Add thyme and celery. Cook 4 minutes. Turn off heat.

2. Remove corn cobs from stock. Add cooked veggies, potatoes, paprika, cayenne, coriander, salt, and pepper. Simmer 25 minutes. Scrape kernels from cobs. Stir in corn kernels and milk. Simmer 3 minutes.

3. Puree 1 quart of soup in a blender until smooth. Return pureed soup to pot. Let simmer, stirring frequently. Hold the bell pepper with tongs over an open flame on the stove. Turn frequently to char all sides.

4. Remove skin, stem, and seeds. Dice bell pepper. Remove soup from heat. Stir in parsley, salt, and pepper. Ladle into bowls and garnish with bell pepper.

## Busting Corn Myths

*Corn is full of healthy nutrients and contains less sugar than an apple. Corn is actually healthier when cooked as more antioxidants get released. Corn is high in fiber.*

# 24. Summer Slaw

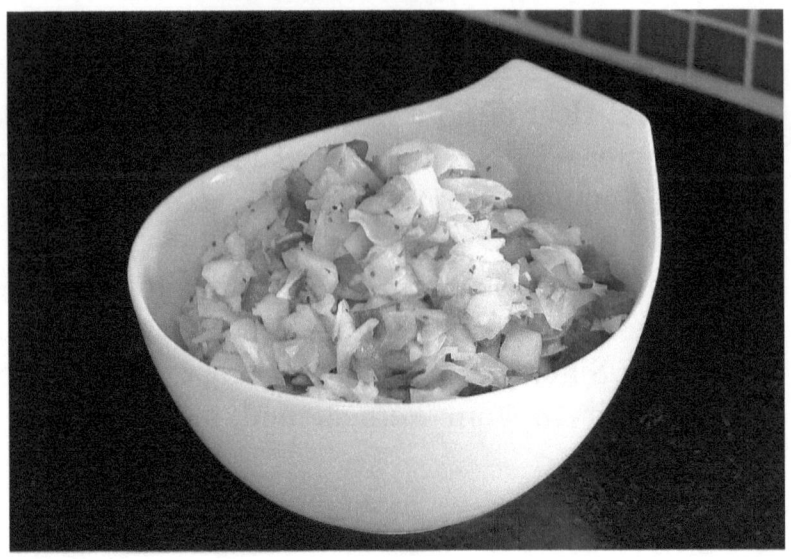

Broccoli turns normal slaw into a deliciously summer experience.

## Ingredients

- 2/3 cup Buttermilk
- 1/3 cup Mayonnaise
- 1 small head Broccoli
- ½ head Cabbage (thinly sliced)
- ½ lbs. Sugar Snap Peas (sliced)
- 4 Tbsps. Chives (chopped)
- 3 Tbsps. Fresh Lemon Juice
- 2 Scallions (sliced)
- Salt & Pepper to taste

## Method

1. In a bowl, whisk together buttermilk, lemon juice, mayonnaise, salt and pepper. Set aside. Halve broccoli pieces lengthwise. Thinly slice crosswise.

2. In a large bowl, toss together broccoli, peas, scallions, cabbage, 2 tablespoons chives, and buttermilk dressing. Season with salt and pepper. Garnish with remaining chives.

## Health Benefits of Broccoli

*Helps lower cholesterol. Helps treat symptoms of allergies. Just ½ a cup of broccoli per day can dramatically lower your risk for cancer.*

# 25. Marinated Summer Veggies

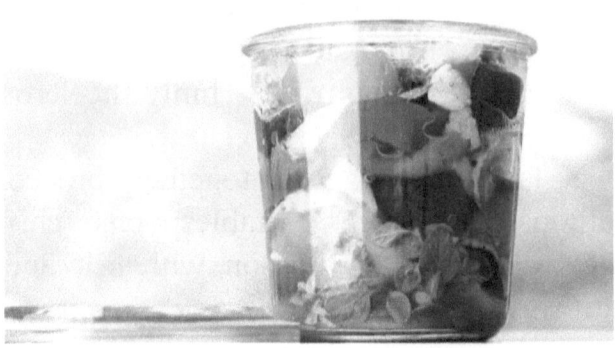

This recipe makes the absolute perfect side dish to a steak or pork chop.

## Ingredients

- 1 lbs. Summer Squash or Zucchini (sliced diagonally)
- 3 Red Bell Peppers (sliced)
- 2 cloves Garlic
- 5 Tbsps. Olive Oil
- 2 Tbsps. Red Wine Vinegar
- 4 sprigs Oregano
- Salt & Pepper to taste

## Method

1. Preheat oven to 475°F. Place squash and peppers each on their own baking sheets. Drizzle 1 tablespoon oil over each. Season with salt and pepper. Toss to coat. Spread out in a single layer.

2. Roast peppers on higher rack in oven. Roast squash on lower rack. Cook 15-20 minutes. Remove skins from peppers.

3. In a bowl, whisk together vinegar, 3 tablespoons oil, garlic, salt and pepper. Add roasted vegetables and oregano. Toss to coat. Cover and let sit 1 hour. Serve.

## Health Benefits of Bell Peppers

*Amazingly high in vitamin A. High in capsaicin which help with weight loss and diabetes. High in lutein and other eye-protecting nutrients.*

# 26. Pan-Fried Summer Squash

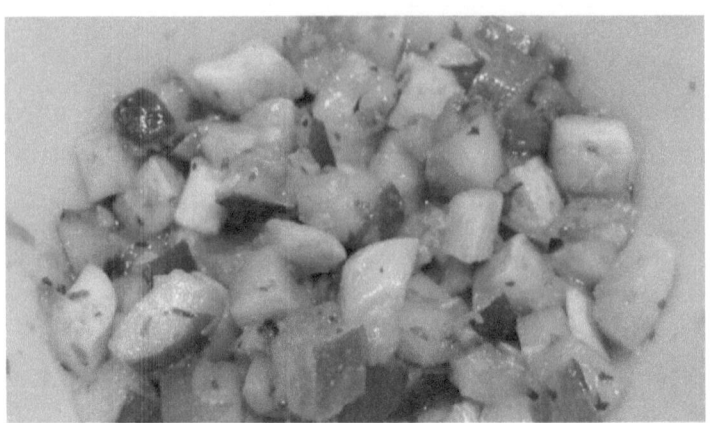

Squash and almonds come together in perfect harmony in this exquisite dish.

## Ingredients

- 2 lbs. Summer Squash or Zucchini (thinly sliced)
- ¼ cup Sliced Almonds
- ¼ cup Parmesan (grated)
- 2 cloves Garlic (sliced)
- 2 Tbsps. Olive Oil
- 1 tsp Crushed Red Pepper Flakes
- Salt & Pepper to taste

## Method

1. In a large bowl, toss squash with 1 teaspoon salt. Let stand 10 minutes. Squeeze squash to remove moisture. Toast almonds in a dry pan on medium heat for 3 minutes. Toss occasionally. Set aside.

2. Heat oil in the same pan over medium heat. Add pepper flakes and garlic. Cook 2 minutes. Add squash. Cook 5 minutes, tossing occasionally. Gradually add in parmesan. Season with salt and pepper. Gradually add in almonds. Serve.

## 3 Ways to Spice up This Dish

*Add chopped jalapeno and lime juice in place of almonds and cheese. Add grated carrot, rice vinegar, and miso instead of cheese. Add cumin and coriander. Dollop with Greek yogurt before serving.*

# 27. Berry Pudding

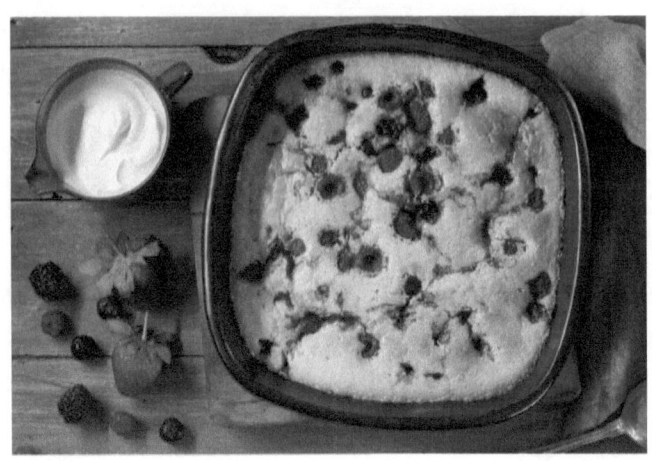

Celebrate the berry season with this simple pudding.

## Ingredients

- 1 (1 lbs.) loaf Brioche or Challah Bread (cut into 1" slices)
- 2 pints Strawberries (quartered)
- 2 pints Blueberries
- 2 pints Blackberries
- 2 pints Raspberries
- 1 cup Sugar
- 1 Vanilla Bean (split lengthwise)
- 6 Tbsps. Butter
- ½ tsp Cinnamon

## Method

1. Line a pan with plastic wrap. Place pan on a baking sheet. In a pot, mix together all berries, ½ cup water,

and 1 cup sugar. Simmer 10 minutes, stirring often. Set aside. Spread butter onto bread slices. Mix 2 tablespoons sugar with cinnamon. Sprinkle over buttered bread.

2. Drizzle ½ cup berry sauce in bottom of lined pan. Arrange a single layer of bread slices in pan. Pour 1 ½ cups berry sauce over bread. Repeat this layering until ingredients are used up. Cover with plastic. Set a plate in the pan and weigh it down with heavy cans. Chill 1 hour.

## Health Benefits of Berries

*Improves brain health and cognitive function. Help control appetite and manage weight. Helps prevent age-related illnesses like Alzheimer's.*

## 28. Corn & Cod Chowder

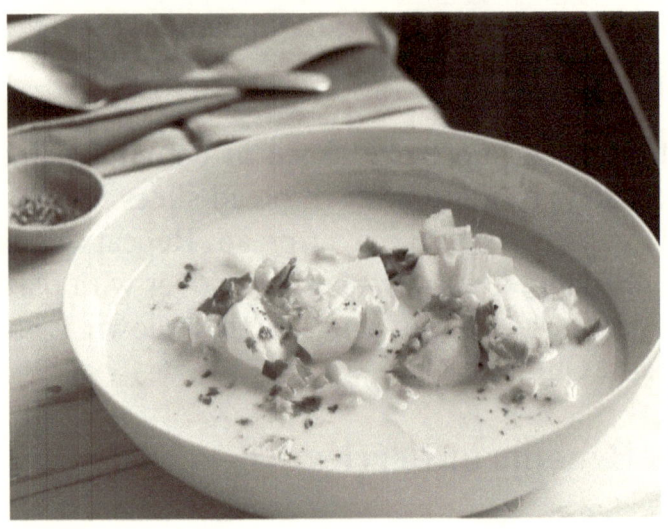

Lighten up a heavy chowder with corn and cod.

## Ingredients

- 3 slices Bacon (Halved)
- 8 Scallions (sliced)
- ¾ lbs. Cod (skin removed, chopped)
- 2 ½ cups Corn Kernels
- ¼ cup Half and Half
- 2 Potatoes (peeled, diced)
- 2 cups Whole Milk
- 2 cups Chicken Broth
- 1 ½ tsp Garlic (chopped)
- 2 Tbsps. Flour
- 2 tsp Thyme
- Salt & Pepper to taste

# Method

1. In a large pan, cook bacon on medium heat for 6 minutes. Let bacon drain on paper towels. Cook scallions in bacon grease 2 minutes. Add garlic. Cook 1 minute. Add flour. Cook 2 minutes, stirring constantly. Stir in milk, broth, potatoes, thyme, salt and pepper. Bring to a boil.

2. Reduce heat to medium-low. Simmer 10 minutes. Stir in cod, corn, and 2 slices of bacon. Simmer 5 minutes. Stir in half and half. Simmer 2 minutes. Crumble remaining slice of bacon. Ladle chowder into bowls. Garnish with bacon crumbles.

## Health Benefits of Cod

*A great low-cholesterol source of protein. High in B vitamins (including the essential B12). High in cholesterol-lowering niacin.*

# 29. Fruit Cobbler

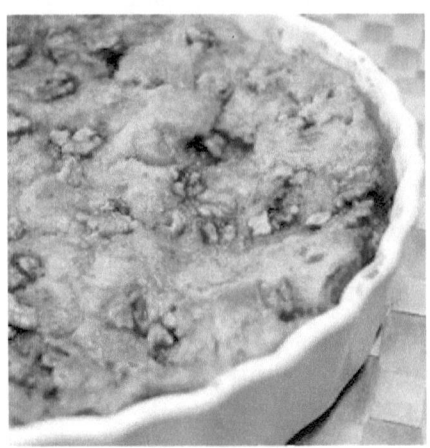

Treat yourself to a summery cobbler with nectarines and raspberries.

## Ingredients

- 4 cups Nectarines (peeled, sliced)
- 1-pint Raspberries
- 2/3 cup Sugar
- 1 ¼ cup Flour
- ½ cup Cornmeal
- 6 Tbsps. Buttermilk
- 5 Tbsps. Butter (sliced)
- 2 Tbsps. Cornstarch
- 1 Tbsp. Raw Sugar
- 1 Tbsp. Fresh Lemon Juice
- 2 tsp Baking Powder
- ¾ tsp Salt
- ½ tsp Baking Soda

## Method

1. Preheat oven to 375°F. In a bowl, toss together raspberries, nectarines, cornstarch, juice, ¼ teaspoon salt, and 1/3 cup sugar. Add mixture to a greased baking dish. In another bowl, whisk together remaining sugar, cornmeal, baking powder, baking soda, flour, and ½ teaspoon salt.

2. Add flour mixture to food processor with butter. Pulse until dough forms pea-sized pieces. Add buttermilk. Pulse until combined. Measure out 1/3 cup portions of dough to create 10 round biscuits. Place biscuits on top of fruit mixture in baking dish. Lightly press biscuits down with fingers. Sprinkle the top with raw sugar. Bake 50 minutes.

## Health Benefits of Nectarines

*High in antioxidants. Helps maintain collagen and prevent wrinkles. Improves digestion and helps weight loss.*

# 30. Summer Stir Fry

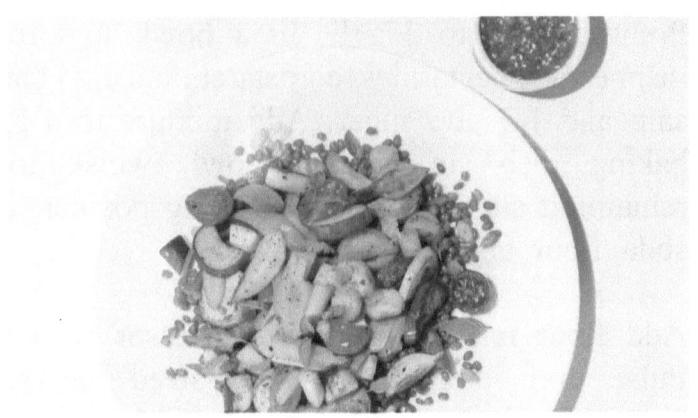

This lively dish is full of bold and vibrant flavors.

## Ingredients

- 4 cups Mixed Summer Veggies (chopped)
- 3 cups Mixed Fresh Herbs (your preference)
- 2 cups Quinoa (cooked)
- ½ cup Scallions (sliced)
- 1 ½" piece Ginger (peeled, sliced)
- 1 clove Garlic
- 7 Tbsps. Olive Oil
- 2 Tbsps. Rice Vinegar
- 2 Tbsps. Sesame Seeds
- Salt & Pepper to taste

## Method

1. Pulse together garlic, ginger, ¼ cup scallions, and 2 cups herbs in a processor. Add 4 tablespoons oil, ¼ cup water, and vinegar. Pulse until pureed. Transfer

to a bowl and stir in sesame seeds. Season with salt and pepper. Heat 1 tablespoon oil in a large pan on medium-high heat.

2. Add remaining scallions and quinoa. Stir fry 3 minutes. Season with salt and pepper. Divide quinoa mix into serving bowls. Return skillet to heat. Add 2 tablespoons oil. Add all vegetables. Season with salt and pepper. Stir fry 4 minutes. Add 1 cup fresh herbs. Toss to combine. Divide vegetable mix into bowls with quinoa. Drizzle herb sauce over the top.

## More Health Benefits of Herbs

*Fresh oregano is a natural anti-inflammatory. Fresh thyme is high in vitamins A & C as well as iron. Fresh sage is the herb with the most antioxidants.*

# 31. Summery Linguine

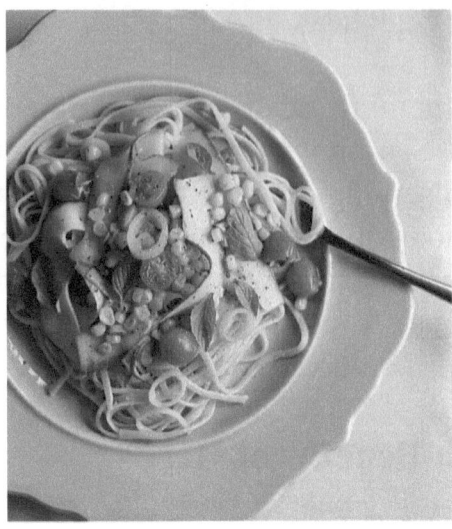

This linguine gets a summer makeover with corn, tomato, and fresh basil.

## Ingredients

- 8 oz. Linguine
- 2 ½ cups Corn Kernels
- 1 ¾ cups Sugar Snap Peas (string-less)
- ½ lbs. Small Tomatoes
- 1 ¼ cup Fresh Basil (chopped)
- ¾ cup Parmesan (grated)
- 3 Tbsps. Olive Oil

## Method

1. Boil linguine until al dente. Drain. Reserve 1 cup of liquid. Place ½ cup liquid in blender. Add ½ cup

corn. Blend until smooth. Heat oil in large pan on medium heat. Add peas and 2 cups corn. Sprinkle in salt and pepper.

2. Cover and cook 5 minutes, stirring often. Add pasta, corn puree, tomatoes, parmesan, and basil. Toss until pasta is thoroughly coated.

## Health Benefits of Snap Peas

*High in vitamin K. High in B vitamins. High in folate.*

# 32. Summer Tarts

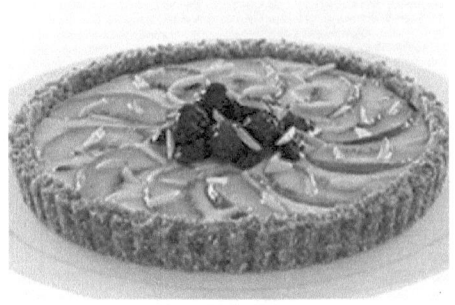

These savory tarts are a great appetizer for a summer barbecue.

## Ingredients

- 2 ½ cups Whole Grain Flour
- 2 sticks Cold Butter (diced)
- 5-8 Tbsps. Water
- ½ tsp Salt
- ¾ cup Whole Milk
- ¾ cup Heavy Cream
- 3 large Eggs
- 1 large Egg Yolk
- 12 Green Beans (trimmed, chopped)
- 12 Grape Tomatoes (halved)
- 6 (¼") slices Goat Cheese
- 2 tsp Chives (chopped)

## Method

1. Blend together butter, salt, and flour in a bowl. Mix with fingers until roughly mixed. Drizzle in 5

tablespoons cold water. Stir with a fork until mixed. If dough doesn't hold together when squeezed, add more cold water ½ tablespoon at a time. Turn dough onto floured surface. Divide into 4 pieces.

2. Press dough out to help distribute butter fat. Gather dough together and form into 2 (5") squares. Wrap in plastic wrap. Chill 1 hour. Arrange 6 flan rings on a baking sheet lined with parchment paper. Roll out chilled dough on a floured surface until it is a 10"x16" rectangle. Cut into 6 squares.

3. Gently fit each pastry square into each flan ring. Trim excess dough so that it is flush with the rim. Gently prick the pastry shells with a fork. Chill 30 minutes. Preheat oven to 375°F. Line shells with foil and place weights in each ring. Bake 20 minutes.

4. Remove weights and foil. Let cool. Reduce oven to 350°F. Boil green beans 3 minutes. Drain and spoon into tart shells. Spoon in tomatoes. Top with round of goat cheese. Whisk together milk, cream, eggs, and egg yolks. Sprinkle in salt and pepper. Divide evenly among tarts. Bake 20 minutes or until custard sets.

## Health Benefits of Whole Grains

*High in both protein and fiber, helping to control appetite and speed up weight loss. Specifically helps reduce belly fat. Help stabilize blood sugar levels.*

# 33. Summer Garden Tortellini

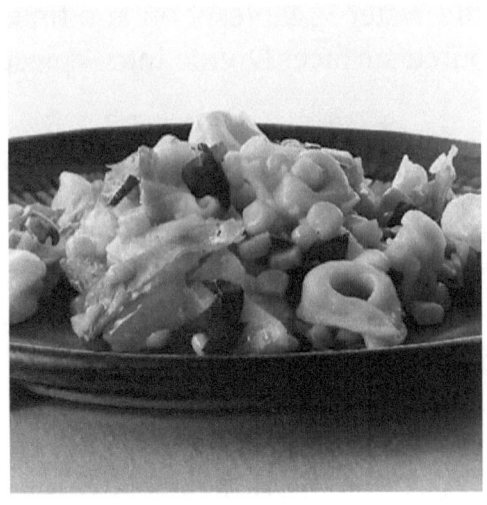

Brighten up your tortellini with the taste of summer.

## Ingredients

- 8 oz. Dried Cheese Tortellini
- 2 cups Corn Kernels
- 2 Tomatoes (chopped)
- 2 oz. Prosciutto Slices (cut into strips)
- 1 clove Garlic (chopped)
- ½ cup Fresh Basil (chopped)
- ½ stick Butter

## Method

1. Cook tortellini in boiling water. In a pan on medium-high heat, cook prosciutto, garlic, butter, salt and pepper 5 minutes.

2. In a large bowl, combine tomatoes with corn mixture. Drain tortellini. Reserve ¼ cup pasta water. Mix tortellini, basil and ¼ cup water in with vegetables. Mix well. Season with salt and pepper.

## Health Benefits of Basil

*Acts as a natural antibacterial. High in vitamin K. High in magnesium and manganese.*

# 34. Summer Kebabs

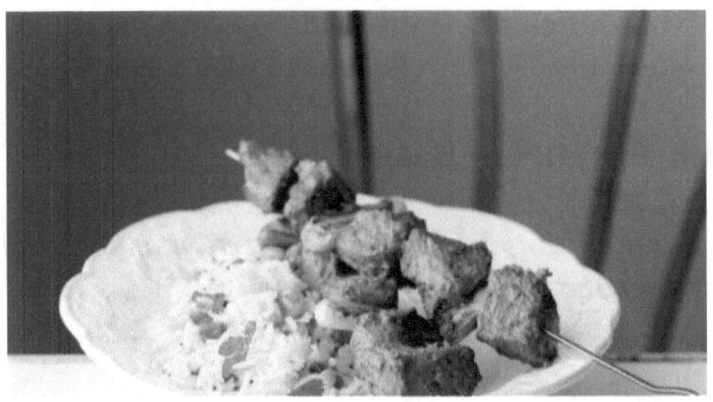

These chicken and summer veggie kebabs come with a fresh salad on the side for a complete summer meal.

## Ingredients

- 5 cups Arugula
- 2 cups Cherry Tomatoes (halved)
- 1 ½ lbs. Boneless Skinless Chicken Breasts (cubed)
- ½ cup Olive Oil
- ¼ cup Balsamic Vinegar
- 1 Red Onion (cut into wedges)
- 2 large Zucchini (cubed)
- 2 Yellow Squash (cubed)
- 1 Orange (juice, zest)
- 1 Lemon (juice, zest)
- 1 Lime (juice, zest)
- 2 tsp Cumin
- 2 tsp Chili Powder
- Pepper to taste

## Method

1. Soak wooden skewers in water 20 minutes. Whisk together ¼ cup oil with the juice and zest from orange, lemon, and lime. Whisk in the cumin and chili powder. Add chicken. Stir to coat. Cover with plastic wrap. Marinate 1 hour.

2. Whisk together ¼ cup oil with vinegar. Coat vegetables with oil-vinegar mixture. Stick the chicken and vegetables onto the skewers in an alternating pattern.

3. Season with pepper. Heat grill to medium-high heat. Cook kebabs about 7 minutes per side (or until chicken is cooked through). Toss arugula with remaining oil-vinegar mixture. Salt and pepper to taste.

## Health Benefits of Olive Oil

*High in unsaturated fats which help you absorb nutrients and stay full for longer. Improves circulation. Can act as a natural pain reliever.*

# 35. Squash Sloppy Joes

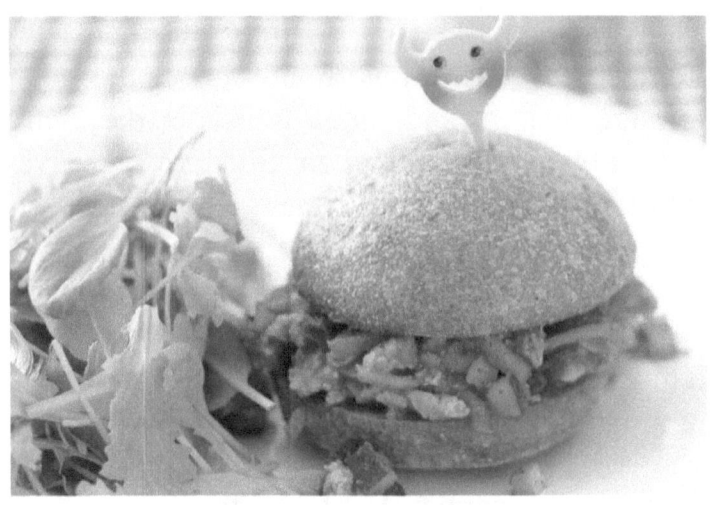

Add new flavors (and more nutritional value) to sloppy joes with this recipe.

## Ingredients

- 6 Hamburger Buns
- 1 lbs. Ground Beef
- 1 ½ cups Summer Squash (diced)
- 1 carrot (chopped)
- ½ Onion (chopped)
- 1 (6oz.) can Tomato Paste
- 3 cloves Garlic (minced)
- 3 oz. Cheddar (sliced)
- 1 Tbsp. Chili Powder
- 1 tsp Paprika
- 1 tsp Oregano
- Salt & Pepper to taste

## Method

1. Preheat broiler. Brown beef in a pan over medium-high heat. Add onion. Cook 2 minutes. Add carrot. Cook 2 minutes. Add squash. Cook 1 minute. Stir in tomato paste and 1 ½ cups water. Stir until dissolved.

2. Add garlic, paprika, chili powder, oregano, salt, and pepper. Reduce heat to medium. Cook 8-10 minutes. Place cheese slices on bottom halves of buns. Toast both sides of buns in broiler (until cheese is melted). Remove buns. Fill sandwiches with meat mixture.

## Health Benefits of Summer Squash

*Lots of lutein and zeaxanthin for eye health. High in tumor-fighting nasunin. High in red blood cell producing B vitamins.*

# 36. Drunken Shaved Ice

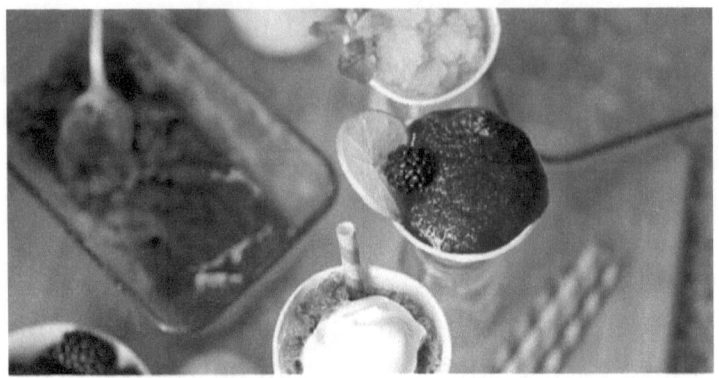

There's no better way to cool off than with spiked shaved ice!

## Ingredients

- 4 cups Shaved Ice
- 1 cup Campari (chilled)

## Method

1. Pack 1 cup shaved ice into each cocktail glass. Drizzle with chilled Campari.

## Try Replacing Campari with:

*A combination of dark rum, apple cider, and lemon juice. Tequila and your favorite margarita mix. A blend of peach nectar, bourbon, mint simple syrup, and lemon juice.*

## 37. Mint Hot Fudge Sundaes

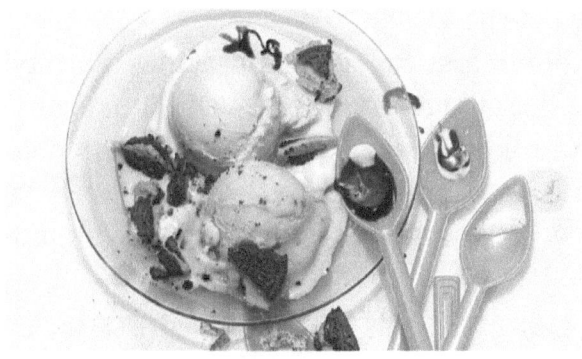

This sundae is soothing and refreshing all at the same time.

## Ingredients

- 1-pint Vanilla Ice Cream
- 1-pint Mint Ice Cream
- 10 Mint Chocolate Oreos (broken)
- 1 cup Dark Chocolate Chunks
- ¼ cup Sugar
- ¼ cup Water
- 1 oz. Unsweetened Chocolate (chopped)
- 2 Tbsps. Fresh Mint
- 1 Tbsp. Sugar
- 2 Tbsps. Butter
- ½ tsp Peppermint Extract
- Sweetened Whipped Cream

## Method

1. In a small pan over medium-high heat, stir together ¼ cup sugar with butter, water, and dark chocolate

chunks. Stir in unsweetened chocolate and peppermint extract until smooth. Set aside.

2. In a bowl, toss together mint and 1 tablespoon sugar. Set aside. Place a scoop of vanilla in each bowl. Top with broken cookies. Scoop in mint ice cream. Top with more cookies. Drizzle the chocolate sauce over. Top with whipped cream. Garnish with mint sugar.

## Health Benefits of Dark Chocolate (70%+ Cacao)

*Contains 11 grams of fiber per 100 grams serving. Rich in antioxidants. High in iron, magnesium, copper, and manganese.*

# 38. Whiskey Wings

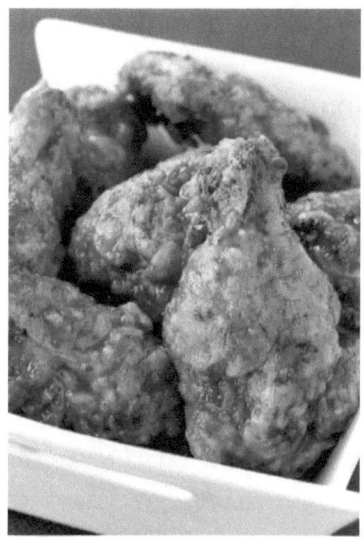

Whiskey adds a new dimension to these scrumptious wings.

## Ingredients

- 24 Chicken Wings
- ¼ cup Dijon Mustard
- ¾ cup BBQ Sauce
- ¼ cup Whiskey
- 1 Tbsp. Sugar
- Salt & Pepper to taste

## Method

1. Cut each wing in half and remove the drumettes. Discard drumettes. Rinse wings well. Pat dry. Season with salt and pepper. Set aside in a Ziploc

bag. In a small pan, whisk together sugar and whiskey. Simmer on medium-high heat. Remove from heat. Whisk in mustard. Cool.

2. Pour the mixture into the bag with the wings. Seal the bag. Toss to coat. Let marinate 30 minutes in the freezer. Prepare the grill for smoking at medium-low heat. Place wings in a shallow aluminum pan. Place pan in grill. Cook 2 hours.

## Health Benefits of Whiskey
*high quality whiskeys in moderation

*Contains heart-healthy antioxidants. May help prevent Alzheimer's and dementia. Helps lower stress.*

# 39. Fruit Salad in Herbed Syrup

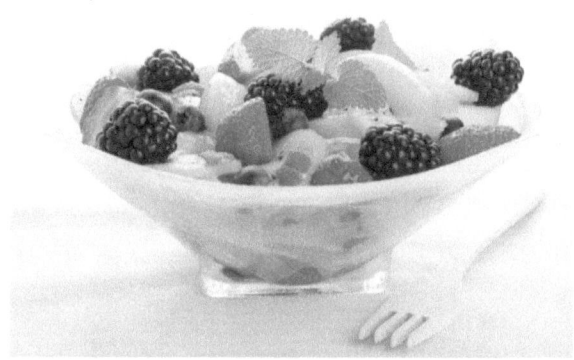

This unique variation on fruit salad is light and refreshing.

## Ingredients

- 1-pint Strawberries (halved)
- ½ pint Raspberries
- ½ pint Blueberries
- 2 Oranges (peeled, sectioned)
- 2 Kiwis (peeled, sliced)
- 1 Mango (peeled, pitted, cubed)
- 1 Papaya (peeled, pitted, cubed)
- 2 cups Pineapple Chunks
- 1 cup Cantaloupe (cubed)
- 1 cup Sugar
- 1 cup Water
- ¼ cup Fresh Rosemary
- ¼ cup Fresh Mint (julienned)
- 1 sprig Rosemary
- 1 sprig Mint

## Method

1. In a small pot, combine 1 cup water, 1 cup sugar, ¼ cup rosemary, and ¼ cup mint. Bring to a boil. Stir until sugar is dissolved. Remove herbs. Set aside.

2. Combine all the fruits into a large bowl. Pour herbed syrup mixture over and mix well. Garnish with rosemary and mint sprigs.

## Health Benefits of Pineapple

*Improves immune system. High in bone-strengthening manganese. Improves gum health.*

# 40. Blueberry Banana Bread

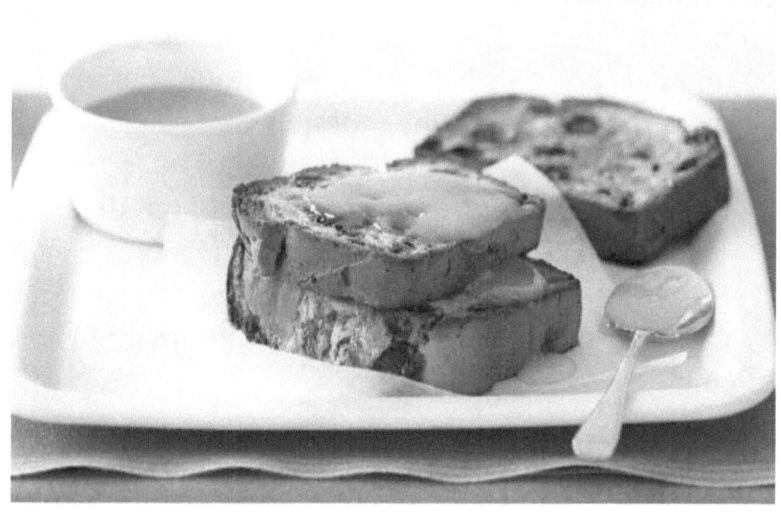

This simple quick bread makes an excellent addition to a relaxing Sunday brunch.

## Ingredients

- ¾ cup Buttermilk
- ¾ cup Brown Sugar
- ¼ cup Olive Oil
- 1 cup Bananas (mashed)
- 2 ¼ cups Whole Grain Flour
- 1 ¼ cup Blueberries
- 2 large Eggs
- ¾ tsp Cinnamon
- 1 ½ tsp Baking Soda
- ¼ tsp Nutmeg
- ½ tsp Salt

## Method

1. Preheat oven to 375°F Whisk together buttermilk, brown sugar, eggs, and oil. Stir in bananas. In another bowl, whisk together flour, baking soda, cinnamon, baking soda, nutmeg, and salt.

2. Stir the dry ingredients into the wet ingredients until combined. Add blueberries. Pour mixture into a greased baking dish. Bake until golden brown and cooked through (about 50 minutes). Cool 10 minutes.

## Health Benefits of Bananas

*Helps treat symptoms of depression. Eaten before workouts, helps prevent muscle cramps. Boost immune system.*

# 41. Frozen Peach Yogurt

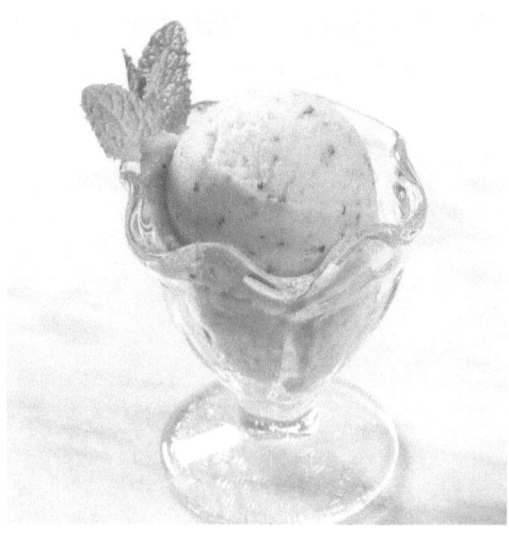

This simple alternative is a great alternative to ice cream on a hot day.

## Ingredients

- 3 ½ cups Frozen Peaches (chopped)
- ½ cup Sugar
- ½ cup Plain Greek Yogurt
- 1 Tbsp. Fresh Lemon Juice

## Method

1. In a food processor, pulse together peaches and sugars. In a bowl, combine yogurt and lemon juice. Pour the yogurt into the processor in batches. Process until smooth and creamy.

## Health Benefits of Peaches

*Helps maintain collagen and moisture in the skin. Helps slow down hair loss and rejuvenate scalp. Helps lower anxiety.*

# Final Words

I would like to thank you for downloading my book and I hope I have been able to help you and educate you about something new.

**If you have enjoyed this book and would like to share your positive thoughts, could you please take 30 seconds of your time to go back and give me a review on my Amazon book page!**

**I greatly appreciate seeing these reviews because it helps me share my hard work!**

Again, thank you and I wish you all the best with your cooking journey!

# Last Chance to Get YOUR Bonus!

**FOR A LIMITED TIME ONLY –** Get Olivia's best-selling book *"The #1 Cookbook: Over 170+ of the Most Popular Recipes Across 7 Different Cuisines!"* absolutely FREE!

Readers have absolutely loved this book because of the wide variety of recipes. It is highly recommended you check these recipes out and see what you can add to your home menu!

Once again, as a big thank-you for downloading this book, I'd like to offer it to you *100% FREE for a LIMITED TIME ONLY!*

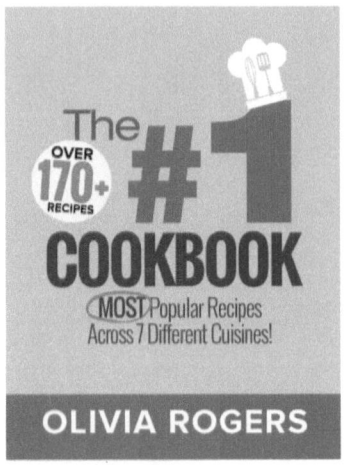

# Get your free copy at:

# TheMenuAtHome.com/Bonus

# Disclaimer

This book and related site provides recipe and food advice in an informative and educational manner only, with information that is general in nature and that is not specific to you, the reader. The contents of this book and related site are intended to assist you and other readers in your personal efforts. Consult your physician or nutritionist regarding the applicability of any information provided in our information to you.

Nothing in this book should be construed as personal advice or diagnosis, and must not be used in this manner. The information provided about conditions is general in nature. This information does not cover all possible uses, actions, precautions, side-effects, or interactions of medicines, or medical procedures. The information in this site should not be considered as complete and does not cover all diseases, ailments, physical conditions, or their treatment.

**No Warranties:** The authors and publishers don't guarantee or warrant the quality, accuracy, completeness, timeliness, appropriateness or suitability of the information in this book, or of any product or services referenced by this site.

The information in this site is provided on an "as is" basis and the authors and publishers make no representations or warranties of any kind with respect to this information.

This site may contain inaccuracies, typographical errors, or other errors.

**Liability Disclaimer:** The publishers, authors, and other parties involved in the creation, production, provision of information, or delivery of this site specifically disclaim any responsibility, and shall not be held liable for any damages, claims, injuries, losses, liabilities, costs, or obligations including any direct, indirect, special, incidental, or consequences damages (collectively known as "Damages") whatsoever and howsoever caused, arising out of, or in connection with the use or misuse of the site and the information contained within it, whether such Damages arise in contract, tort, negligence, equity, statute law, or by way of other legal theory.

www.ingramcontent.com/pod-product-compliance
Lightning Source LLC
Chambersburg PA
CBHW021129080526
44587CB00012B/1199